GET
YOUR
KETO
ON

90-DAY KETO DIET PLANNER &
WEIGHT LOSS JOURNAL

THIS JOURNAL BELONGS TO:

_____

Name

MY JOURNEY STARTS ON:

_____

Date

LETTER FROM THE FOUNDERS

Welcome!

We are so happy to have you here and are super excited to see you start this journey to a healthier you!

Just a little background about the faces behind this KETO journal, my husband and I are the co-founders of RIMSports! We created this brand of sporting goods and accessories because of our shared love for fitness and for each other (yes, cheesy I know).

It all started four years ago when we decided to workout at our local gym after struggling with failed diets and fluctuating weight gain. We both desperately needed to improve our health because of a history of illness in our families and the damaging habits we were creating for ourselves and future generations.

Because it had been a while since we visited a gym, I wanted to match my workout gloves with my outfit (because doesn't everyone)! Failing to find any vibrant colors other than black, Colin found a way to make a pair of pink gloves and surprised me with the first ever RIMSports Weightlifting Gloves.

Over the years, we as a small-family business have made the values of hard work, vision, and focus our guiding principles. We spend every waking moment creating higher quality and more durable products for our customers that we would be confident to use and proud to wear.

After talking with industry experts, fitness trainers, body-builders, and our loyal customers, we have devised an all-encompassing way to KETO meals and macros, alongside your weight loss goals. There is no comparable KETO guide on the market that lets you record your macros next to your meals!

You see, we are just like you! We've struggled with our inability to stick to our daily meal plans and schedules. This is why we created this journal - to stay accountable. We hope you find value in not only our story but this KETO journal, as you take this bold step toward your weight-loss goals and living your best life!

Ever humbly yours,

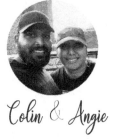

Colin & Angie

CROSS A BIG "X"

OVER EACH DAY YOU COMPLETE YOUR DAILY GOALS

1	2	3	4	5	6	7	8	9	10
11	12	13	14	15	16	17	18	19	20
21	22	23	24	25	26	27	28	29	30
31	32	33	34	35	36	37	38	39	40
41	42	43	44	45	46	47	48	49	50
51	52	53	54	55	56	57	58	59	60
61	62	63	64	65	66	67	68	69	70
71	72	73	74	75	76	77	78	79	80
81	82	83	84	85	86	87	88	89	90

D A Y S

30 DAYS

Break
Unhealty
Habits!

60 DAYS

Celebrate
Your
Progress!

90 DAYS

Enjoy
Your
Success!

BODY MEASUREMENTS

MEASUREMENT GUIDE

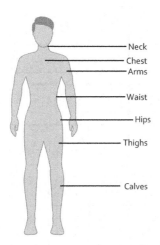

- Neck
- Chest
- Arms
- Waist
- Hips
- Thighs
- Calves

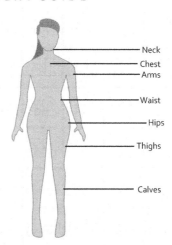

- Neck
- Chest
- Arms
- Waist
- Hips
- Thighs
- Calves

PROGRESS TRACKER

	Today	Week 1	Week 2	Week 3	Week 4	Week 5	Week 6	Week 7	Week 8	Week 9	Week 10	Week 11	Week 12	Week 13
Neck														
Chest														
Arms														
Waist														
Hips														
Thighs														
Calves														
Weight														
Body Fat														
Other														

TIPS
Use a flexible measuring tape, such as plastic or cloth.

When taking measurements, stand tall with your muscles relaxed and feet together.

TIPS
Apply constant pressure to the tape (so it doesn't sag) without pinching the skin.

Measure under the same conditions each time, such as wearing the same clothes (or none at all).

TIPS
Measure yourself in front of a mirror to make sure the tape is positioned correctly. If possible, have someone else do the measuring for you.

How I feel today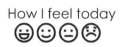

DAY 1

Had cravings today

*"In this moment
I feel peaceful and content"*

MY GOALS

Date:

FOOD	BREAKFAST	LUNCH	DINNER	SNACKS
	_____	_____	_____	_____
	_____	_____	_____	_____
	_____	_____	_____	_____
	_____	_____	_____	_____
	CALORIES :	CALORIES :	CALORIES :	CALORIES :

MACROS			WEIGHTS & REPS
	FATS		
	CARBS		
	PROTEINS		

FITNESS	WATER INTAKE	CALORIES	SLEEP TIME	WAKE TIME	WEIGHT
MIN / HRS	▢▢▢▢▢▢▢▢				

NON-SCALE VICTORIES	

How I feel today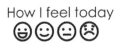

DAY
2

Had cravings today

*"I am worthy of all the best life
has to offer."*

MY GOALS

Date:

	BREAKFAST	LUNCH	DINNER	SNACKS
FOOD	_____	_____	_____	_____
	_____	_____	_____	_____
	_____	_____	_____	_____
	_____	_____	_____	_____
	CALORIES :	CALORIES :	CALORIES :	CALORIES :

			WEIGHTS & REPS
MACROS	**FATS**		
	CARBS		
	PROTEINS		

FITNESS	WATER INTAKE	CALORIES	SLEEP TIME	WAKE TIME	WEIGHT
MIN / HRS	🥛🥛🥛🥛🥛🥛🥛🥛				

NON-SCALE VICTORIES	

How I feel today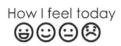

DAY 3

Had cravings today

"I release all resistance to feeling good."

MY GOALS

Date:

FOOD	BREAKFAST	LUNCH	DINNER	SNACKS
	CALORIES :	CALORIES :	CALORIES :	CALORIES :

MACROS	FATS		WEIGHTS & REPS
	CARBS		
	PROTEINS		

FITNESS	WATER INTAKE	CALORIES	SLEEP TIME	WAKE TIME	WEIGHT
MIN / HRS					

NON-SCALE VICTORIES	

How I feel today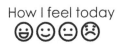

DAY 4

Had cravings today

"Ieven in the midst of chaos
I can always maintain my inner peace."

MY GOALS

Date:

	BREAKFAST	LUNCH	DINNER	SNACKS
FOOD				
	CALORIES :	CALORIES :	CALORIES :	CALORIES :

MACROS	FATS		WEIGHTS & REPS
	CARBS		
	PROTEINS		

FITNESS	WATER INTAKE	CALORIES	SLEEP TIME	WAKE TIME	WEIGHT
MIN / HRS					

NON-SCALE VICTORIES	

How I feel today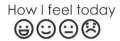

DAY 5

Had cravings today

*"I am always free to choose, and today
I choose happiness."*

MY GOALS

Date:

	BREAKFAST	LUNCH	DINNER	SNACKS
FOOD				
	CALORIES :	CALORIES :	CALORIES :	CALORIES :

			WEIGHTS & REPS
MACROS	**FATS**		
	CARBS		
	PROTEINS		

FITNESS	WATER INTAKE	CALORIES	SLEEP TIME	WAKE TIME	WEIGHT
MIN / HRS					

NON-SCALE VICTORIES	

How I feel today Had cravings today

😀 ☺ 😐 😖   Ⓨ Ⓝ

"I am open to new and exciting possibilities."

MY GOALS

Date:

	BREAKFAST	LUNCH	DINNER	SNACKS
FOOD				
	CALORIES :	CALORIES :	CALORIES :	CALORIES :

MACROS	FATS		WEIGHTS & REPS
	CARBS		
	PROTEINS		

FITNESS	WATER INTAKE	CALORIES	SLEEP TIME	WAKE TIME	WEIGHT
MIN / HRS					

NON-SCALE VICTORIES	

How I feel today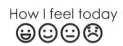

Had cravings today

"I attract pleasant, positive people into my life."

MY GOALS

Date:

FOOD	BREAKFAST	LUNCH	DINNER	SNACKS
	___	___	___	___
	___	___	___	___
	___	___	___	___
	___	___	___	___
	CALORIES :	CALORIES :	CALORIES :	CALORIES :

MACROS	FATS		WEIGHTS & REPS
	CARBS		
	PROTEINS		

FITNESS	WATER INTAKE	CALORIES	SLEEP TIME	WAKE TIME	WEIGHT
MIN / HRS	🥛🥛🥛🥛🥛🥛🥛🥛				

NON-SCALE VICTORIES	

WEEKLY CHECK-IN

CHECK IN

	M	T	W	T	F	S	S
Drink 8 glasses water	☐	☐	☐	☐	☐	☐	☐
Take my vitamins / supplements	☐	☐	☐	☐	☐	☐	☐
Recorded in my food journal	☐	☐	☐	☐	☐	☐	☐
Measured my weight	☐	☐	☐	☐	☐	☐	☐
Take my electrolytes	☐	☐	☐	☐	☐	☐	☐
Made fat bombs	☐	☐	☐	☐	☐	☐	☐

MEAL PLAN

- _____
- _____
- _____
- _____
- _____
- _____

DID YOU ACCOMPLISH LAST WEEK'S GOALS? IF NOT, WHY?

_____

_____

_____

NEXT WEEK'S GOALS

How I feel today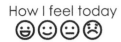

Had cravings today

"I am enjoying the life I'm living."

MY GOALS

Date:

FOOD	BREAKFAST	LUNCH	DINNER	SNACKS
	_____	_____	_____	_____
	_____	_____	_____	_____
	_____	_____	_____	_____
	_____	_____	_____	_____
	CALORIES :	CALORIES :	CALORIES :	CALORIES :

MACROS	FATS		WEIGHTS & REPS
	CARBS		
	PROTEINS		

FITNESS	WATER INTAKE	CALORIES	SLEEP TIME	WAKE TIME	WEIGHT
MIN / HRS					

	NON-SCALE VICTORIES

How I feel today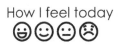

Had cravings today

"I have fun and laugh every day."

MY GOALS

Date:

FOOD	BREAKFAST	LUNCH	DINNER	SNACKS
	_____ _____ _____ _____	_____ _____ _____ _____	_____ _____ _____ _____	_____ _____ _____ _____
	CALORIES :	CALORIES :	CALORIES :	CALORIES :

MACROS	FATS		WEIGHTS & REPS
	CARBS		
	PROTEINS		

FITNESS	WATER INTAKE	CALORIES	SLEEP TIME	WAKE TIME	WEIGHT
MIN / HRS					

NON-SCALE VICTORIES	

How I feel today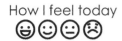

Had cravings today

"I experience joy and create joy for others."

MY GOALS

Date:

FOOD	BREAKFAST	LUNCH	DINNER	SNACKS
	_____	_____	_____	_____
	_____	_____	_____	_____
	_____	_____	_____	_____
	_____	_____	_____	_____
	CALORIES :	CALORIES :	CALORIES :	CALORIES :

MACROS	FATS		WEIGHTS & REPS
	CARBS		
	PROTEINS		

FITNESS	WATER INTAKE	CALORIES	SLEEP TIME	WAKE TIME	WEIGHT
MIN / HRS	🥛🥛🥛🥛🥛🥛🥛🥛				

NON-SCALE VICTORIES	

How I feel today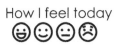

 DAY 11

Had cravings today

"Each morning I wake up feeling enthusiastic about the day ahead."

MY GOALS

Date:

	BREAKFAST	LUNCH	DINNER	SNACKS
FOOD	———— ———— ———— ———— ———— ———— ———— ————	———— ———— ———— ———— ———— ———— ———— ————	———— ———— ———— ———— ———— ———— ———— ————	———— ———— ———— ———— ———— ———— ———— ————
	CALORIES :	CALORIES :	CALORIES :	CALORIES :

MACROS	FATS		WEIGHTS & REPS
	CARBS		
	PROTEINS		

FITNESS	WATER INTAKE	CALORIES	SLEEP TIME	WAKE TIME	WEIGHT
MIN / HRS	🥤🥤🥤🥤🥤🥤🥤🥤				

NON-SCALE VICTORIES	

How I feel today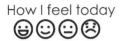

DAY
12

Had cravings today

*"Each night I go to sleep feeling fulfilled,
thankful, and peaceful."*

MY GOALS

Date:

	BREAKFAST	LUNCH	DINNER	SNACKS
FOOD				
	CALORIES :	CALORIES :	CALORIES :	CALORIES :

			WEIGHTS & REPS
MACROS	**FATS**		
	CARBS		
	PROTEINS		

FITNESS	WATER INTAKE	CALORIES	SLEEP TIME	WAKE TIME	WEIGHT
MIN / HRS					

NON-SCALE VICTORIES	

How I feel today Had cravings today

😀 ☺ 😐 😣   Ⓨ Ⓝ

"I always look for the good in everyone around me."

MY GOALS

Date:

FOOD	BREAKFAST	LUNCH	DINNER	SNACKS
	_____	_____	_____	_____
	_____	_____	_____	_____
	_____	_____	_____	_____
	_____	_____	_____	_____
	CALORIES :	CALORIES :	CALORIES :	CALORIES :

MACROS	FATS		WEIGHTS & REPS
	CARBS		
	PROTEINS		

FITNESS	WATER INTAKE	CALORIES	SLEEP TIME	WAKE TIME	WEIGHT
MIN / HRS	🥛🥛🥛🥛🥛🥛🥛🥛				

NON-SCALE VICTORIES

How I feel today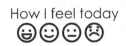

DAY 14

Had cravings today

"I appreciate all the positive people in my life."

MY GOALS

Date:

FOOD	BREAKFAST	LUNCH	DINNER	SNACKS
	_____	_____	_____	_____
	_____	_____	_____	_____
	_____	_____	_____	_____
	_____	_____	_____	_____
	CALORIES :	CALORIES :	CALORIES :	CALORIES :

MACROS	FATS		WEIGHTS & REPS
	CARBS		
	PROTEINS		

FITNESS	WATER INTAKE	CALORIES	SLEEP TIME	WAKE TIME	WEIGHT
MIN / HRS					

NON-SCALE VICTORIES	

WEEKLY CHECK-IN

CHECK IN

	M	T	W	T	F	S	S
Drink 8 glasses water	☐	☐	☐	☐	☐	☐	☐
Take my vitamins / supplements	☐	☐	☐	☐	☐	☐	☐
Recorded in my food journal	☐	☐	☐	☐	☐	☐	☐
Measured my weight	☐	☐	☐	☐	☐	☐	☐
Take my electrolytes	☐	☐	☐	☐	☐	☐	☐
Made fat bombs	☐	☐	☐	☐	☐	☐	☐

MEAL PLAN

- _____
- _____
- _____

- _____
- _____
- _____

DID YOU ACCOMPLISH LAST WEEK'S GOALS? IF NOT, WHY?

_____

_____

_____

NEXT WEEK'S GOALS

How I feel today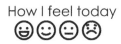

DAY 15

Had cravings today

*"I have wonderful friends, and we all help
and support each other."*

MY GOALS

Date:

FOOD	BREAKFAST	LUNCH	DINNER	SNACKS
	_____	_____	_____	_____
	_____	_____	_____	_____
	_____	_____	_____	_____
	_____	_____	_____	_____
	CALORIES :	CALORIES :	CALORIES :	CALORIES :

MACROS	FATS		WEIGHTS & REPS
	CARBS		
	PROTEINS		

FITNESS	WATER INTAKE	CALORIES	SLEEP TIME	WAKE TIME	WEIGHT
MIN / HRS	🥤🥤🥤🥤🥤🥤🥤🥤				

NON-SCALE VICTORIES

How I feel today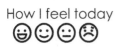

DAY
16

Had cravings today

"I feel healthy, fit, and strong."

MY GOALS

Date:

	BREAKFAST	LUNCH	DINNER	SNACKS
FOOD				
	CALORIES :	CALORIES :	CALORIES :	CALORIES :

			WEIGHTS & REPS
MACROS	**FATS**		
	CARBS		
	PROTEINS		

FITNESS	WATER INTAKE	CALORIES	SLEEP TIME	WAKE TIME	WEIGHT
MIN / HRS					

NON-SCALE VICTORIES	

How I feel today
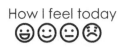

 DAY 17

Had cravings today

"I have abundant energy."

MY GOALS

Date:

	BREAKFAST	LUNCH	DINNER	SNACKS
FOOD				
	CALORIES :	CALORIES :	CALORIES :	CALORIES :

			WEIGHTS & REPS
MACROS	**FATS**		
	CARBS		
	PROTEINS		

FITNESS	WATER INTAKE	CALORIES	SLEEP TIME	WAKE TIME	WEIGHT
MIN / HRS					

NON-SCALE VICTORIES	

How I feel today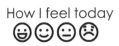

DAY 18

Had cravings today

"I effortlessly attract health, wealth,
happiness, and love."

MY GOALS

Date:

FOOD	BREAKFAST	LUNCH	DINNER	SNACKS
	————	————	————	————
	————	————	————	————
	————	————	————	————
	————	————	————	————
	CALORIES :	CALORIES :	CALORIES :	CALORIES :

MACROS	FATS		WEIGHTS & REPS
	CARBS		
	PROTEINS		

FITNESS	WATER INTAKE	CALORIES	SLEEP TIME	WAKE TIME	WEIGHT
MIN / HRS	🥛🥛🥛🥛🥛🥛🥛🥛				

NON-SCALE VICTORIES	

How I feel today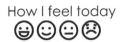

DAY 19

Had cravings today

*"My joyful, peaceful energy is a blessing
to those around me."*

MY GOALS

Date:

FOOD	BREAKFAST	LUNCH	DINNER	SNACKS
	————	————	————	————
	————	————	————	————
	————	————	————	————
	————	————	————	————
	CALORIES :	CALORIES :	CALORIES :	CALORIES :

MACROS	FATS		WEIGHTS & REPS
	CARBS		
	PROTEINS		

FITNESS	WATER INTAKE	CALORIES	SLEEP TIME	WAKE TIME	WEIGHT
MIN / HRS	🥛🥛🥛🥛🥛🥛🥛🥛				

NON-SCALE VICTORIES

How I feel today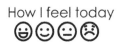

Had cravings today

*"I am happy, joyous and free, exactly
as I was born to be."*

MY GOALS

Date:

FOOD	BREAKFAST	LUNCH	DINNER	SNACKS
	_____	_____	_____	_____
	_____	_____	_____	_____
	_____	_____	_____	_____
	_____	_____	_____	_____
	CALORIES :	CALORIES :	CALORIES :	CALORIES :

MACROS	FATS		WEIGHTS & REPS
	CARBS		
	PROTEINS		

FITNESS	WATER INTAKE	CALORIES	SLEEP TIME	WAKE TIME	WEIGHT
MIN / HRS	🥛🥛🥛🥛🥛🥛🥛🥛				

NON-SCALE VICTORIES	

How I feel today Had cravings today

😄 😊 😐 😣

"I let go of all fear, resistance, and barriers to love."

MY GOALS

Date:

FOOD	BREAKFAST	LUNCH	DINNER	SNACKS
	CALORIES :	CALORIES :	CALORIES :	CALORIES :

MACROS	FATS		WEIGHTS & REPS
	CARBS		
	PROTEINS		

FITNESS	WATER INTAKE	CALORIES	SLEEP TIME	WAKE TIME	WEIGHT
MIN / HRS	🥛🥛🥛🥛🥛🥛🥛				

NON-SCALE VICTORIES

WEEKLY CHECK-IN

CHECK IN

	M	T	W	T	F	S	S
Drink 8 glasses water	☐	☐	☐	☐	☐	☐	☐
Take my vitamins / supplements	☐	☐	☐	☐	☐	☐	☐
Recorded in my food journal	☐	☐	☐	☐	☐	☐	☐
Measured my weight	☐	☐	☐	☐	☐	☐	☐
Take my electrolytes	☐	☐	☐	☐	☐	☐	☐
Made fat bombs	☐	☐	☐	☐	☐	☐	☐

MEAL PLAN

-
-
-
-
-
-

DID YOU ACCOMPLISH LAST WEEK'S GOALS? IF NOT, WHY?

NEXT WEEK'S GOALS

How I feel today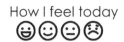

Had cravings today

"I love myself as I love others."

MY GOALS

Date:

	BREAKFAST	LUNCH	DINNER	SNACKS
FOOD				
	CALORIES :	CALORIES :	CALORIES :	CALORIES :

			WEIGHTS & REPS
MACROS	**FATS**		
	CARBS		
	PROTEINS		

FITNESS	WATER INTAKE	CALORIES	SLEEP TIME	WAKE TIME	WEIGHT
MIN / HRS					

NON-SCALE VICTORIES	

How I feel today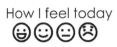

Had cravings today

"I am worthy of all the love the universe has to offer me."

MY GOALS

Date:

FOOD	BREAKFAST	LUNCH	DINNER	SNACKS
	CALORIES :	CALORIES :	CALORIES :	CALORIES :

MACROS	FATS		WEIGHTS & REPS
	CARBS		
	PROTEINS		

FITNESS	WATER INTAKE	CALORIES	SLEEP TIME	WAKE TIME	WEIGHT
MIN / HRS					

NON-SCALE VICTORIES

How I feel today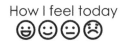

Had cravings today

*"I enjoy loving relationships with
my friends and my family members."*

MY GOALS

Date:

	BREAKFAST	LUNCH	DINNER	SNACKS
FOOD				
	CALORIES :	CALORIES :	CALORIES :	CALORIES :

			WEIGHTS & REPS
MACROS	FATS		
	CARBS		
	PROTEINS		

FITNESS	WATER INTAKE	CALORIES	SLEEP TIME	WAKE TIME	WEIGHT
MIN / HRS	🥛🥛🥛🥛🥛🥛🥛🥛				

NON-SCALE VICTORIES	

How I feel today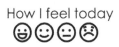

Had cravings today

"My heart is open to all the love that surrounds me."

MY GOALS

Date:

FOOD	BREAKFAST	LUNCH	DINNER	SNACKS
	_____	_____	_____	_____
	_____	_____	_____	_____
	_____	_____	_____	_____
	_____	_____	_____	_____
	CALORIES :	CALORIES :	CALORIES :	CALORIES :

MACROS	FATS		WEIGHTS & REPS
	CARBS		
	PROTEINS		

FITNESS	WATER INTAKE	CALORIES	SLEEP TIME	WAKE TIME	WEIGHT
MIN / HRS	🥛🥛🥛🥛🥛🥛🥛🥛				

NON-SCALE VICTORIES

How I feel today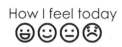

DAY 26

Had cravings today

"Love fills my life in abundance every day."

MY GOALS

Date:

FOOD	BREAKFAST	LUNCH	DINNER	SNACKS
	_____	_____	_____	_____
	_____	_____	_____	_____
	_____	_____	_____	_____
	_____	_____	_____	_____
	CALORIES :	CALORIES :	CALORIES :	CALORIES :

MACROS	FATS		WEIGHTS & REPS
	CARBS		
	PROTEINS		

FITNESS	WATER INTAKE	CALORIES	SLEEP TIME	WAKE TIME	WEIGHT
MIN / HRS					

NON-SCALE VICTORIES	

How I feel today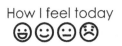

Had cravings today

"I know the joy of giving and receiving unconditional love."

MY GOALS

Date:

FOOD	BREAKFAST	LUNCH	DINNER	SNACKS
	_____	_____	_____	_____
	_____	_____	_____	_____
	_____	_____	_____	_____
	_____	_____	_____	_____
	CALORIES :	CALORIES :	CALORIES :	CALORIES :

MACROS	FATS		WEIGHTS & REPS
	CARBS		
	PROTEINS		

FITNESS	WATER INTAKE	CALORIES	SLEEP TIME	WAKE TIME	WEIGHT
MIN / HRS					

NON-SCALE VICTORIES	

How I feel today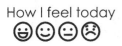

Had cravings today

*"I am attracting more and more
loving relationships into my life."*

MY GOALS

Date:

FOOD	BREAKFAST	LUNCH	DINNER	SNACKS
	_____	_____	_____	_____
	_____	_____	_____	_____
	_____	_____	_____	_____
	_____	_____	_____	_____
	CALORIES :	CALORIES :	CALORIES :	CALORIES :

MACROS	FATS		WEIGHTS & REPS
	CARBS		
	PROTEINS		

FITNESS	WATER INTAKE	CALORIES	SLEEP TIME	WAKE TIME	WEIGHT
MIN / HRS					

NON-SCALE VICTORIES	

WEEKLY CHECK-IN

CHECK IN

	M	T	W	T	F	S	S
Drink 8 glasses water	☐	☐	☐	☐	☐	☐	☐
Take my vitamins / supplements	☐	☐	☐	☐	☐	☐	☐
Recorded in my food journal	☐	☐	☐	☐	☐	☐	☐
Measured my weight	☐	☐	☐	☐	☐	☐	☐
Take my electrolytes	☐	☐	☐	☐	☐	☐	☐
Made fat bombs	☐	☐	☐	☐	☐	☐	☐

MEAL PLAN

- _____
- _____
- _____
- _____
- _____
- _____

DID YOU ACCOMPLISH LAST WEEK'S GOALS? IF NOT, WHY?

NEXT WEEK'S GOALS

How I feel today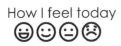

DAY
29

Had cravings today

*"As I seek the love of my life,
the love of my life is seeking me."*

MY GOALS

Date:

FOOD	BREAKFAST	LUNCH	DINNER	SNACKS
	_____	_____	_____	_____
	_____	_____	_____	_____
	_____	_____	_____	_____
	_____	_____	_____	_____
	CALORIES :	CALORIES :	CALORIES :	CALORIES :

MACROS	FATS		WEIGHTS & REPS
	CARBS		
	PROTEINS		

FITNESS	WATER INTAKE	CALORIES	SLEEP TIME	WAKE TIME	WEIGHT
MIN / HRS	🥛🥛🥛🥛🥛🥛🥛				

NON-SCALE VICTORIES

How I feel today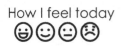

Had cravings today
(Y) (N)

"I am grateful for the love and romance that I am attracting."

MY GOALS

Date:

	BREAKFAST	LUNCH	DINNER	SNACKS
FOOD				
	CALORIES :	CALORIES :	CALORIES :	CALORIES :

MACROS	FATS		WEIGHTS & REPS
	CARBS		
	PROTEINS		

FITNESS	WATER INTAKE	CALORIES	SLEEP TIME	WAKE TIME	WEIGHT
MIN / HRS	🥛🥛🥛🥛🥛🥛🥛🥛				

NON-SCALE VICTORIES

How I feel today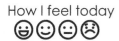

DAY
31

Had cravings today

"I think, speak, and act from the place within me that is love."

MY GOALS

Date:

FOOD	BREAKFAST	LUNCH	DINNER	SNACKS
	CALORIES :	CALORIES :	CALORIES :	CALORIES :

MACROS	FATS		WEIGHTS & REPS
	CARBS		
	PROTEINS		

FITNESS	WATER INTAKE	CALORIES	SLEEP TIME	WAKE TIME	WEIGHT
MIN / HRS					

NON-SCALE VICTORIES	

How I feel today
😃 😊 😐 😞

DAY 32

Had cravings today
Ⓨ Ⓝ

"The more love I give, the more I receive."

MY GOALS

Date:

	BREAKFAST	LUNCH	DINNER	SNACKS
FOOD				
	CALORIES :	CALORIES :	CALORIES :	CALORIES :

MACROS	FATS		WEIGHTS & REPS
	CARBS		
	PROTEINS		

FITNESS	WATER INTAKE	CALORIES	SLEEP TIME	WAKE TIME	WEIGHT
MIN / HRS	🥛🥛🥛🥛🥛🥛🥛				

NON-SCALE VICTORIES	

How I feel today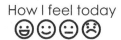

Had cravings today

*"I am spending time with a person
who accepts me just as I am."*

MY GOALS

Date:

	BREAKFAST	LUNCH	DINNER	SNACKS
FOOD	_____	_____	_____	_____
	_____	_____	_____	_____
	_____	_____	_____	_____
	_____	_____	_____	_____
	CALORIES :	CALORIES :	CALORIES :	CALORIES :

			WEIGHTS & REPS
MACROS	**FATS**		
	CARBS		
	PROTEINS		

FITNESS	WATER INTAKE	CALORIES	SLEEP TIME	WAKE TIME	WEIGHT
MIN / HRS	🥛🥛🥛🥛🥛🥛🥛🥛				

NON-SCALE VICTORIES	

How I feel today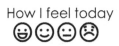

Had cravings today

*"My new partner and I enjoy laughing together
and finding new ways to have fun."*

MY GOALS

Date:

	BREAKFAST	LUNCH	DINNER	SNACKS
FOOD				
	CALORIES :	CALORIES :	CALORIES :	CALORIES :

			WEIGHTS & REPS
MACROS	**FATS**		
	CARBS		
	PROTEINS		

FITNESS	WATER INTAKE	CALORIES	SLEEP TIME	WAKE TIME	WEIGHT
MIN / HRS					

NON-SCALE VICTORIES	

How I feel today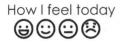

Had cravings today

*"My new partner and I know the joy of
mutual love, trust, and respect."*

MY GOALS

Date:

FOOD	BREAKFAST	LUNCH	DINNER	SNACKS
	CALORIES :	CALORIES :	CALORIES :	CALORIES :

MACROS	FATS		WEIGHTS & REPS
	CARBS		
	PROTEINS		

FITNESS	WATER INTAKE	CALORIES	SLEEP TIME	WAKE TIME	WEIGHT
MIN / HRS					

NON-SCALE VICTORIES

WEEKLY CHECK-IN

CHECK IN

	M	T	W	T	F	S	S
Drink 8 glasses water	☐	☐	☐	☐	☐	☐	☐
Take my vitamins / supplements	☐	☐	☐	☐	☐	☐	☐
Recorded in my food journal	☐	☐	☐	☐	☐	☐	☐
Measured my weight	☐	☐	☐	☐	☐	☐	☐
Take my electrolytes	☐	☐	☐	☐	☐	☐	☐
Made fat bombs	☐	☐	☐	☐	☐	☐	☐

MEAL PLAN

- _____
- _____
- _____

- _____
- _____
- _____

DID YOU ACCOMPLISH LAST WEEK'S GOALS? IF NOT, WHY?

NEXT WEEK'S GOALS

How I feel today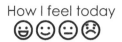

Had cravings today

(Y) (N)

"I welcome the passion and romance flowing into my life."

Date:

MY GOALS

	BREAKFAST	LUNCH	DINNER	SNACKS
FOOD				
	CALORIES :	CALORIES :	CALORIES :	CALORIES :

			WEIGHTS & REPS
MACROS	FATS		
	CARBS		
	PROTEINS		

FITNESS	WATER INTAKE	CALORIES	SLEEP TIME	WAKE TIME	WEIGHT
MIN / HRS					

NON-SCALE VICTORIES

How I feel today
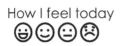

DAY
37

Had cravings today

Y   N

*"Emotional intimacy is a natural,
daily part of my relationship."*

MY GOALS

Date:

FOOD	BREAKFAST	LUNCH	DINNER	SNACKS
	_____	_____	_____	_____
	_____	_____	_____	_____
	_____	_____	_____	_____
	_____	_____	_____	_____
	CALORIES :	CALORIES :	CALORIES :	CALORIES :

MACROS	FATS		WEIGHTS & REPS
	CARBS		
	PROTEINS		

FITNESS	WATER INTAKE	CALORIES	SLEEP TIME	WAKE TIME	WEIGHT
MIN / HRS	🥛🥛🥛🥛🥛🥛🥛🥛				

NON-SCALE VICTORIES

How I feel today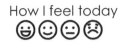

DAY
38

Had cravings today

"All conflict in my relationship is resolved calmly and respectfully."

MY GOALS

Date:

FOOD	BREAKFAST	LUNCH	DINNER	SNACKS
	————	————	————	————
	————	————	————	————
	————	————	————	————
	————	————	————	————
	CALORIES :	CALORIES :	CALORIES :	CALORIES :

MACROS	FATS		WEIGHTS & REPS
	CARBS		
	PROTEINS		

FITNESS	WATER INTAKE	CALORIES	SLEEP TIME	WAKE TIME	WEIGHT
MIN / HRS	🥛🥛🥛🥛🥛🥛🥛🥛				

NON-SCALE VICTORIES	

How I feel today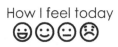

DAY 39

Had cravings today

"I have healthy boundaries, and I feel safe and secure."

MY GOALS

Date:

	BREAKFAST	LUNCH	DINNER	SNACKS
FOOD				
	CALORIES :	CALORIES :	CALORIES :	CALORIES :

			WEIGHTS & REPS
MACROS	**FATS**		
	CARBS		
	PROTEINS		

FITNESS	WATER INTAKE	CALORIES	SLEEP TIME	WAKE TIME	WEIGHT
MIN / HRS					

NON-SCALE VICTORIES

How I feel today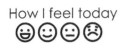

Had cravings today

(Y) (N)

"Every day my relationship grows stronger,
and our love grows deeper."

MY GOALS

Date:

FOOD	BREAKFAST	LUNCH	DINNER	SNACKS
	————	————	————	————
	————	————	————	————
	————	————	————	————
	————	————	————	————
	CALORIES :	CALORIES :	CALORIES :	CALORIES :

MACROS	FATS		WEIGHTS & REPS
	CARBS		
	PROTEINS		

FITNESS	WATER INTAKE	CALORIES	SLEEP TIME	WAKE TIME	WEIGHT
MIN / HRS					

NON-SCALE VICTORIES	

How I feel today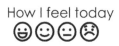

Had cravings today

(Y) (N)

"I am blessed with a partner who is truly my soul mate."

MY GOALS

Date:

FOOD	BREAKFAST	LUNCH	DINNER	SNACKS
	_____	_____	_____	_____
	_____	_____	_____	_____
	_____	_____	_____	_____
	_____	_____	_____	_____
	CALORIES :	CALORIES :	CALORIES :	CALORIES :

MACROS	FATS		WEIGHTS & REPS
	CARBS		
	PROTEINS		

FITNESS	WATER INTAKE	CALORIES	SLEEP TIME	WAKE TIME	WEIGHT
MIN / HRS	🥛🥛🥛🥛🥛🥛🥛🥛				

NON-SCALE VICTORIES

How I feel today

😃 ☺ 😐 😞

DAY 42

Had cravings today

Ⓨ Ⓝ

"I accept me just as I am."

MY GOALS

Date:

FOOD	BREAKFAST	LUNCH	DINNER	SNACKS
	CALORIES :	CALORIES :	CALORIES :	CALORIES :

MACROS	FATS		WEIGHTS & REPS
	CARBS		
	PROTEINS		

FITNESS	WATER INTAKE	CALORIES	SLEEP TIME	WAKE TIME	WEIGHT
MIN / HRS	🥛🥛🥛🥛🥛🥛🥛🥛				

NON-SCALE VICTORIES	

WEEKLY CHECK-IN

CHECK IN

	M	T	W	T	F	S	S
Drink 8 glasses water	☐	☐	☐	☐	☐	☐	☐
Take my vitamins / supplements	☐	☐	☐	☐	☐	☐	☐
Recorded in my food journal	☐	☐	☐	☐	☐	☐	☐
Measured my weight	☐	☐	☐	☐	☐	☐	☐
Take my electrolytes	☐	☐	☐	☐	☐	☐	☐
Made fat bombs	☐	☐	☐	☐	☐	☐	☐

MEAL PLAN

- _____
- _____
- _____
- _____
- _____
- _____

DID YOU ACCOMPLISH LAST WEEK'S GOALS? IF NOT, WHY?

_____

_____

_____

NEXT WEEK'S GOALS

How I feel today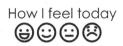

Had cravings today

"I am a loving, compassionate, and giving person."

MY GOALS

Date:

FOOD	BREAKFAST	LUNCH	DINNER	SNACKS
	CALORIES :	CALORIES :	CALORIES :	CALORIES :

MACROS	FATS		WEIGHTS & REPS
	CARBS		
	PROTEINS		

FITNESS	WATER INTAKE	CALORIES	SLEEP TIME	WAKE TIME	WEIGHT
MIN / HRS					

NON-SCALE VICTORIES

How I feel today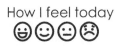

DAY 44

Had cravings today

*"I am worthy, and my heart is open
to receiving love."*

MY GOALS

Date:

	BREAKFAST	LUNCH	DINNER	SNACKS
FOOD				
	CALORIES :	CALORIES :	CALORIES :	CALORIES :

			WEIGHTS & REPS
MACROS	**FATS**		
	CARBS		
	PROTEINS		

FITNESS	WATER INTAKE	CALORIES	SLEEP TIME	WAKE TIME	WEIGHT
MIN / HRS					

NON-SCALE VICTORIES	

How I feel today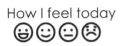

 DAY 45

Had cravings today

*"I forgive myself and others
fully and completely."*

MY GOALS

Date:

FOOD	BREAKFAST	LUNCH	DINNER	SNACKS
	_____	_____	_____	_____
	_____	_____	_____	_____
	_____	_____	_____	_____
	_____	_____	_____	_____
	CALORIES :	CALORIES :	CALORIES :	CALORIES :

MACROS	FATS		WEIGHTS & REPS
	CARBS		
	PROTEINS		

FITNESS	WATER INTAKE	CALORIES	SLEEP TIME	WAKE TIME	WEIGHT
MIN / HRS					

NON-SCALE VICTORIES

How I feel today

DAY 46

Had cravings today

"I peacefully let go of past thoughts and feelings that no longer serve me."

MY GOALS

Date:

FOOD	BREAKFAST	LUNCH	DINNER	SNACKS
	————	————	————	————
	————	————	————	————
	————	————	————	————
	————	————	————	————
	CALORIES :	CALORIES :	CALORIES :	CALORIES :

MACROS	FATS		WEIGHTS & REPS
	CARBS		
	PROTEINS		

FITNESS	WATER INTAKE	CALORIES	SLEEP TIME	WAKE TIME	WEIGHT
MIN / HRS	🥛🥛🥛🥛🥛🥛🥛🥛				

NON-SCALE VICTORIES	

How I feel today

Had cravings today

DAY 47

"I see my family through the eyes of love."

MY GOALS

Date:

	BREAKFAST	LUNCH	DINNER	SNACKS
FOOD	_____	_____	_____	_____
	_____	_____	_____	_____
	_____	_____	_____	_____
	CALORIES :	CALORIES :	CALORIES :	CALORIES :

MACROS	FATS		WEIGHTS & REPS
	CARBS		
	PROTEINS		

FITNESS	WATER INTAKE	CALORIES	SLEEP TIME	WAKE TIME	WEIGHT
MIN / HRS					

NON-SCALE VICTORIES	

How I feel today 😃 😊 😐 😖

Had cravings today

Ⓨ Ⓝ

"I am grateful for every member of my family."

MY GOALS

Date:

	BREAKFAST	LUNCH	DINNER	SNACKS
FOOD				
	CALORIES :	CALORIES :	CALORIES :	CALORIES :

MACROS	FATS		WEIGHTS & REPS
	CARBS		
	PROTEINS		

FITNESS	WATER INTAKE	CALORIES	SLEEP TIME	WAKE TIME	WEIGHT
MIN / HRS	🥛🥛🥛🥛🥛🥛🥛🥛				

NON-SCALE VICTORIES	

How I feel today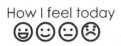

DAY 49

Had cravings today

(Y) (N)

"I accept my family members just as they are."

MY GOALS

Date:

FOOD	BREAKFAST	LUNCH	DINNER	SNACKS
	_____	_____	_____	_____
	_____	_____	_____	_____
	_____	_____	_____	_____
	_____	_____	_____	_____
	CALORIES :	CALORIES :	CALORIES :	CALORIES :

MACROS	FATS		WEIGHTS & REPS
	CARBS		
	PROTEINS		

FITNESS	WATER INTAKE	CALORIES	SLEEP TIME	WAKE TIME	WEIGHT
MIN / HRS	🥛🥛🥛🥛🥛🥛🥛🥛				

NON-SCALE VICTORIES	

WEEKLY CHECK-IN

CHECK IN

	M	T	W	T	F	S	S
Drink 8 glasses water	☐	☐	☐	☐	☐	☐	☐
Take my vitamins / supplements	☐	☐	☐	☐	☐	☐	☐
Recorded in my food journal	☐	☐	☐	☐	☐	☐	☐
Measured my weight	☐	☐	☐	☐	☐	☐	☐
Take my electrolytes	☐	☐	☐	☐	☐	☐	☐
Made fat bombs	☐	☐	☐	☐	☐	☐	☐

MEAL PLAN

- _____
- _____
- _____
- _____
- _____
- _____

DID YOU ACCOMPLISH LAST WEEK'S GOALS? IF NOT, WHY?

_____

_____

_____

NEXT WEEK'S GOALS

How I feel today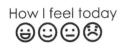

Had cravings today

"I am grateful that my family accepts me for who I am."

MY GOALS

Date:

	BREAKFAST	LUNCH	DINNER	SNACKS
FOOD				
	CALORIES :	CALORIES :	CALORIES :	CALORIES :

MACROS	FATS		WEIGHTS & REPS
	CARBS		
	PROTEINS		

FITNESS	WATER INTAKE	CALORIES	SLEEP TIME	WAKE TIME	WEIGHT
MIN / HRS					

NON-SCALE VICTORIES	

How I feel today Had cravings today

😃 🙂 😐 😣 (Y) (N)

"Every day I send the energy of love, light, and
happiness to each member of my family."

MY GOALS

Date:

	BREAKFAST	LUNCH	DINNER	SNACKS
FOOD	_____	_____	_____	_____
	_____	_____	_____	_____
	_____	_____	_____	_____
	_____	_____	_____	_____
	CALORIES :	CALORIES :	CALORIES :	CALORIES :

			WEIGHTS & REPS
MACROS	**FATS**		
	CARBS		
	PROTEINS		

FITNESS	WATER INTAKE	CALORIES	SLEEP TIME	WAKE TIME	WEIGHT
MIN / HRS	🥛🥛🥛🥛🥛🥛🥛🥛				

NON-SCALE VICTORIES	

How I feel today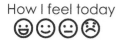

DAY 52

Had cravings today

"All the relationships in my life are blessed with healing love."

MY GOALS

Date:

	BREAKFAST	LUNCH	DINNER	SNACKS
FOOD				
	CALORIES :	CALORIES :	CALORIES :	CALORIES :

			WEIGHTS & REPS
MACROS	**FATS**		
	CARBS		
	PROTEINS		

FITNESS	WATER INTAKE	CALORIES	SLEEP TIME	WAKE TIME	WEIGHT
MIN / HRS					

NON-SCALE VICTORIES

How I feel today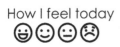

Had cravings today

"In the presence of my family I feel safe,
peaceful, and content."

MY GOALS

Date:

	BREAKFAST	LUNCH	DINNER	SNACKS
FOOD	————	————	————	————
	————	————	————	————
	————	————	————	————
	————	————	————	————
	CALORIES :	CALORIES :	CALORIES :	CALORIES :

			WEIGHTS & REPS
MACROS	**FATS**		
	CARBS		
	PROTEINS		

FITNESS	WATER INTAKE	CALORIES	SLEEP TIME	WAKE TIME	WEIGHT
MIN / HRS	🥤🥤🥤🥤🥤🥤🥤🥤				

NON-SCALE VICTORIES

How I feel today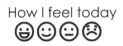

DAY 54

Had cravings today

"My family and I communicate
with each other freely and openly."

MY GOALS

Date:

	BREAKFAST	LUNCH	DINNER	SNACKS
FOOD	_____	_____	_____	_____
	_____	_____	_____	_____
	_____	_____	_____	_____
	_____	_____	_____	_____
	CALORIES :	CALORIES :	CALORIES :	CALORIES :

			WEIGHTS & REPS
MACROS	**FATS**		
	CARBS		
	PROTEINS		

FITNESS	WATER INTAKE	CALORIES	SLEEP TIME	WAKE TIME	WEIGHT
MIN / HRS	🥛🥛🥛🥛🥛🥛🥛🥛				

NON-SCALE VICTORIES	

How I feel today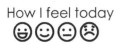

Had cravings today

*"My family members always respond to
each other's concerns with compassion and support."*

MY GOALS

Date:

BREAKFAST	LUNCH	DINNER	SNACKS
FOOD			
CALORIES :	CALORIES :	CALORIES :	CALORIES :

MACROS	FATS		WEIGHTS & REPS
	CARBS		
	PROTEINS		

FITNESS	WATER INTAKE	CALORIES	SLEEP TIME	WAKE TIME	WEIGHT
MIN / HRS					

NON-SCALE VICTORIES

How I feel today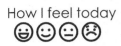

DAY
56

Had cravings today

"I love my children unconditionally."

MY GOALS

Date:

	BREAKFAST	LUNCH	DINNER	SNACKS
FOOD				
	CALORIES :	CALORIES :	CALORIES :	CALORIES :

			WEIGHTS & REPS
MACROS	**FATS**		
	CARBS		
	PROTEINS		

FITNESS	WATER INTAKE	CALORIES	SLEEP TIME	WAKE TIME	WEIGHT
MIN / HRS					

NON-SCALE VICTORIES	

WEEKLY CHECK-IN

CHECK IN

	M	T	W	T	F	S	S
Drink 8 glasses water	☐	☐	☐	☐	☐	☐	☐
Take my vitamins / supplements	☐	☐	☐	☐	☐	☐	☐
Recorded in my food journal	☐	☐	☐	☐	☐	☐	☐
Measured my weight	☐	☐	☐	☐	☐	☐	☐
Take my electrolytes	☐	☐	☐	☐	☐	☐	☐
Made fat bombs	☐	☐	☐	☐	☐	☐	☐

MEAL PLAN

- _____
- _____
- _____
- _____
- _____
- _____

DID YOU ACCOMPLISH LAST WEEK'S GOALS? IF NOT, WHY?

_____

_____

_____

NEXT WEEK'S GOALS

How I feel today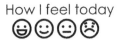

DAY
57

Had cravings today

"I tell my children I love them and show them through my actions."

MY GOALS

Date:

FOOD	BREAKFAST	LUNCH	DINNER	SNACKS
	_____	_____	_____	_____
	_____	_____	_____	_____
	_____	_____	_____	_____
	_____	_____	_____	_____
	CALORIES :	CALORIES :	CALORIES :	CALORIES :

MACROS	FATS		WEIGHTS & REPS
	CARBS		
	PROTEINS		

FITNESS	WATER INTAKE	CALORIES	SLEEP TIME	WAKE TIME	WEIGHT
MIN / HRS	🥛🥛🥛🥛🥛🥛🥛🥛				

NON-SCALE VICTORIES	

How I feel today

DAY 58

Had cravings today

"I am a patient, understanding, and supportive parent."

MY GOALS

Date:

	BREAKFAST	LUNCH	DINNER	SNACKS
FOOD				
	CALORIES :	CALORIES :	CALORIES :	CALORIES :

			WEIGHTS & REPS
MACROS	**FATS**		
	CARBS		
	PROTEINS		

FITNESS	WATER INTAKE	CALORIES	SLEEP TIME	WAKE TIME	WEIGHT
MIN / HRS					

NON-SCALE VICTORIES	

How I feel today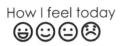

DAY 59

Had cravings today

*"I empower my children by being
a positive role model."*

<u>**MY GOALS**</u>

Date:

FOOD	BREAKFAST	LUNCH	DINNER	SNACKS
	————	————	————	————
	————	————	————	————
	————	————	————	————
	————	————	————	————
	CALORIES :	CALORIES :	CALORIES :	CALORIES :

MACROS	FATS		WEIGHTS & REPS
	CARBS		
	PROTEINS		

FITNESS	WATER INTAKE	CALORIES	SLEEP TIME	WAKE TIME	WEIGHT
MIN / HRS					

NON-SCALE VICTORIES	

How I feel today Had cravings today

😆 ☺ 😐 😣

DAY 60

"I delight in each little joy my children share with me."

MY GOALS

Date:

FOOD	BREAKFAST	LUNCH	DINNER	SNACKS
	———	———	———	———
	———	———	———	———
	———	———	———	———
	———	———	———	———
	CALORIES :	CALORIES :	CALORIES :	CALORIES :

MACROS	FATS		WEIGHTS & REPS
	CARBS		
	PROTEINS		

FITNESS	WATER INTAKE	CALORIES	SLEEP TIME	WAKE TIME	WEIGHT
MIN / HRS	🥛🥛🥛🥛🥛🥛🥛🥛				

NON-SCALE VICTORIES	

How I feel today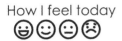

Had cravings today

"My children are happy, healthy, and thriving."

MY GOALS

Date:

	BREAKFAST	LUNCH	DINNER	SNACKS
FOOD				
	CALORIES :	CALORIES :	CALORIES :	CALORIES :

			WEIGHTS & REPS
MACROS	**FATS**		
	CARBS		
	PROTEINS		

FITNESS	WATER INTAKE	CALORIES	SLEEP TIME	WAKE TIME	WEIGHT
MIN / HRS					

NON-SCALE VICTORIES

How I feel today

DAY 62

Had cravings today

Ⓨ Ⓝ

"I let go of all urges to criticize myself."

MY GOALS

Date:

	BREAKFAST	LUNCH	DINNER	SNACKS
FOOD				
	CALORIES :	CALORIES :	CALORIES :	CALORIES :

			WEIGHTS & REPS
MACROS	**FATS**		
	CARBS		
	PROTEINS		

FITNESS	WATER INTAKE	CALORIES	SLEEP TIME	WAKE TIME	WEIGHT
MIN / HRS	🥛🥛🥛🥛🥛🥛🥛🥛				

NON-SCALE VICTORIES	

How I feel today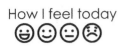

Had cravings today

"I accept me and approve of me exactly as I am."

MY GOALS

Date:

FOOD	BREAKFAST	LUNCH	DINNER	SNACKS
	_____	_____	_____	_____
	_____	_____	_____	_____
	_____	_____	_____	_____
	_____	_____	_____	_____
	CALORIES :	CALORIES :	CALORIES :	CALORIES :

MACROS	FATS		WEIGHTS & REPS
	CARBS		
	PROTEINS		

FITNESS	WATER INTAKE	CALORIES	SLEEP TIME	WAKE TIME	WEIGHT
MIN / HRS					

NON-SCALE VICTORIES	

WEEKLY CHECK-IN

CHECK IN

	M	T	W	T	F	S	S
Drink 8 glasses water	☐	☐	☐	☐	☐	☐	☐
Take my vitamins / supplements	☐	☐	☐	☐	☐	☐	☐
Recorded in my food journal	☐	☐	☐	☐	☐	☐	☐
Measured my weight	☐	☐	☐	☐	☐	☐	☐
Take my electrolytes	☐	☐	☐	☐	☐	☐	☐
Made fat bombs	☐	☐	☐	☐	☐	☐	☐

MEAL PLAN

- _____
- _____
- _____
- _____
- _____
- _____

DID YOU ACCOMPLISH LAST WEEK'S GOALS? IF NOT, WHY?

_____

_____

_____

NEXT WEEK'S GOALS

How I feel today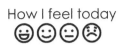

DAY 64

Had cravings today

*" I have a good mind, a kind heart,
and a gentle spirit. "*

MY GOALS

Date:

FOOD	BREAKFAST	LUNCH	DINNER	SNACKS
	_____	_____	_____	_____
	_____	_____	_____	_____
	_____	_____	_____	_____
	_____	_____	_____	_____
	CALORIES :	CALORIES :	CALORIES :	CALORIES :

MACROS	FATS		WEIGHTS & REPS
	CARBS		
	PROTEINS		

FITNESS	WATER INTAKE	CALORIES	SLEEP TIME	WAKE TIME	WEIGHT
MIN / HRS					

NON-SCALE VICTORIES

How I feel today

DAY 65

Had cravings today
(Y) (N)

"I believe in myself."

MY GOALS

Date:

FOOD	BREAKFAST	LUNCH	DINNER	SNACKS
	_____	_____	_____	_____
	_____	_____	_____	_____
	_____	_____	_____	_____
	_____	_____	_____	_____
	CALORIES :	CALORIES :	CALORIES :	CALORIES :

MACROS	FATS		WEIGHTS & REPS
	CARBS		
	PROTEINS		

FITNESS	WATER INTAKE	CALORIES	SLEEP TIME	WAKE TIME	WEIGHT
MIN / HRS	🥤🥤🥤🥤🥤🥤🥤				

NON-SCALE VICTORIES	

How I feel today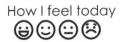

DAY
66

Had cravings today
(Y) (N)

"I am strong, confident, and powerful."

MY GOALS

Date:

FOOD	BREAKFAST	LUNCH	DINNER	SNACKS
	_____	_____	_____	_____
	_____	_____	_____	_____
	_____	_____	_____	_____
	_____	_____	_____	_____
	CALORIES :	CALORIES :	CALORIES :	CALORIES :

MACROS	FATS		WEIGHTS & REPS
	CARBS		
	PROTEINS		

FITNESS	WATER INTAKE	CALORIES	SLEEP TIME	WAKE TIME	WEIGHT
MIN / HRS					

NON-SCALE VICTORIES

How I feel today Had cravings today

"I am a beautiful human being, inside and out."

MY GOALS

Date:

	BREAKFAST	LUNCH	DINNER	SNACKS
FOOD				
	CALORIES :	CALORIES :	CALORIES :	CALORIES :

			WEIGHTS & REPS
MACROS	**FATS**		
	CARBS		
	PROTEINS		

FITNESS	WATER INTAKE	CALORIES	SLEEP TIME	WAKE TIME	WEIGHT
MIN / HRS					

NON-SCALE VICTORIES	

How I feel today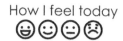

DAY 68

Had cravings today

"I am intelligent, capable, and competent."

Date:

MY GOALS

FOOD	BREAKFAST	LUNCH	DINNER	SNACKS
	CALORIES :	CALORIES :	CALORIES :	CALORIES :

MACROS	FATS		WEIGHTS & REPS
	CARBS		
	PROTEINS		

FITNESS	WATER INTAKE	CALORIES	SLEEP TIME	WAKE TIME	WEIGHT
MIN / HRS					

NON-SCALE VICTORIES

How I feel today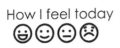

Had cravings today

"I see each new challenge as an opportunity to grow."

MY GOALS

Date:

	BREAKFAST	LUNCH	DINNER	SNACKS
FOOD				
	CALORIES :	CALORIES :	CALORIES :	CALORIES :

MACROS	FATS		WEIGHTS & REPS
	CARBS		
	PROTEINS		

FITNESS	WATER INTAKE	CALORIES	SLEEP TIME	WAKE TIME	WEIGHT
MIN / HRS					

NON-SCALE VICTORIES	

How I feel today Had cravings today

DAY 70

(Y) (N)

*"I trust myself, and I make decisions
with ease and confidence."*

MY GOALS

Date:

	BREAKFAST	LUNCH	DINNER	SNACKS
FOOD				
	CALORIES :	CALORIES :	CALORIES :	CALORIES :

			WEIGHTS & REPS
MACROS	**FATS**		
	CARBS		
	PROTEINS		

FITNESS	WATER INTAKE	CALORIES	SLEEP TIME	WAKE TIME	WEIGHT
MIN / HRS					

NON-SCALE VICTORIES	

WEEKLY CHECK-IN

CHECK IN

	M	T	W	T	F	S	S
Drink 8 glasses water	☐	☐	☐	☐	☐	☐	☐
Take my vitamins / supplements	☐	☐	☐	☐	☐	☐	☐
Recorded in my food journal	☐	☐	☐	☐	☐	☐	☐
Measured my weight	☐	☐	☐	☐	☐	☐	☐
Take my electrolytes	☐	☐	☐	☐	☐	☐	☐
Made fat bombs	☐	☐	☐	☐	☐	☐	☐

MEAL PLAN

- _____
- _____
- _____
- _____
- _____
- _____

DID YOU ACCOMPLISH LAST WEEK'S GOALS? IF NOT, WHY?

_____

_____

_____

NEXT WEEK'S GOALS

How I feel today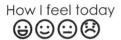

DAY 71

Had cravings today

"I am free from all negative beliefs from my past."

MY GOALS

Date:

	BREAKFAST	LUNCH	DINNER	SNACKS
FOOD				
	CALORIES :	CALORIES :	CALORIES :	CALORIES :

			WEIGHTS & REPS
MACROS	**FATS**		
	CARBS		
	PROTEINS		

FITNESS	WATER INTAKE	CALORIES	SLEEP TIME	WAKE TIME	WEIGHT
MIN / HRS					

NON-SCALE VICTORIES	

How I feel today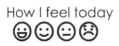

 DAY 72

Had cravings today

"I am learning to step out of my comfort zone without fear."

MY GOALS

Date:

FOOD	BREAKFAST	LUNCH	DINNER	SNACKS
	_____	_____	_____	_____
	_____	_____	_____	_____
	_____	_____	_____	_____
	_____	_____	_____	_____
	CALORIES :	CALORIES :	CALORIES :	CALORIES :

MACROS	FATS		WEIGHTS & REPS
	CARBS		
	PROTEINS		

FITNESS	WATER INTAKE	CALORIES	SLEEP TIME	WAKE TIME	WEIGHT
MIN / HRS	🥛🥛🥛🥛🥛🥛🥛🥛				

NON-SCALE VICTORIES

How I feel today

How I feel today 😃 🙂 😐 ☹️

DAY
73

Had cravings today

Ⓨ Ⓝ

"I have the courage to live in the truth of who I am."

MY GOALS

Date:

FOOD	BREAKFAST	LUNCH	DINNER	SNACKS
	_____	_____	_____	_____
	_____	_____	_____	_____
	_____	_____	_____	_____
	_____	_____	_____	_____
	CALORIES :	CALORIES :	CALORIES :	CALORIES :

MACROS	FATS		WEIGHTS & REPS
	CARBS		
	PROTEINS		

FITNESS	WATER INTAKE	CALORIES	SLEEP TIME	WAKE TIME	WEIGHT
MIN / HRS	🥛🥛🥛🥛🥛🥛🥛🥛				

NON-SCALE VICTORIES	

How I feel today

😃 ☺ 😐 ☹

 DAY **74**

Had cravings today

Ⓨ Ⓝ

"I am completely open to new experiences."

MY GOALS

Date:

FOOD	BREAKFAST	LUNCH	DINNER	SNACKS
	————	————	————	————
	————	————	————	————
	————	————	————	————
	————	————	————	————
	CALORIES :	CALORIES :	CALORIES :	CALORIES :

MACROS	FATS		WEIGHTS & REPS
	CARBS		
	PROTEINS		

FITNESS	WATER INTAKE	CALORIES	SLEEP TIME	WAKE TIME	WEIGHT
MIN / HRS	🥛🥛🥛🥛🥛🥛🥛				

NON-SCALE VICTORIES	

How I feel today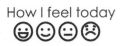

DAY
75

Had cravings today

*"I recognize mistakes as stepping stones
to learning and honing my skills."*

MY GOALS

Date:

FOOD	BREAKFAST	LUNCH	DINNER	SNACKS
	_____	_____	_____	_____
	CALORIES :	CALORIES :	CALORIES :	CALORIES :

MACROS	FATS		WEIGHTS & REPS
	CARBS		
	PROTEINS		

FITNESS	WATER INTAKE	CALORIES	SLEEP TIME	WAKE TIME	WEIGHT
MIN / HRS					

NON-SCALE VICTORIES	

How I feel today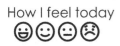

Had cravings today

*"My energy and enthusiasm for life
increases every day."*

MY GOALS

Date:

	BREAKFAST	LUNCH	DINNER	SNACKS
FOOD				
	CALORIES :	CALORIES :	CALORIES :	CALORIES :

			WEIGHTS & REPS
MACROS	**FATS**		
	CARBS		
	PROTEINS		

FITNESS	WATER INTAKE	CALORIES	SLEEP TIME	WAKE TIME	WEIGHT
MIN / HRS					

NON-SCALE VICTORIES	

How I feel today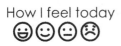

Had cravings today

*"I have faith in myself and trust
my inner wisdom to guide me."*

MY GOALS

Date:

	BREAKFAST	LUNCH	DINNER	SNACKS
FOOD				
	CALORIES :	CALORIES :	CALORIES :	CALORIES :

			WEIGHTS & REPS
MACROS	**FATS**		
	CARBS		
	PROTEINS		

FITNESS	WATER INTAKE	CALORIES	SLEEP TIME	WAKE TIME	WEIGHT
MIN / HRS					

NON-SCALE VICTORIES

WEEKLY CHECK-IN

CHECK IN

	M	T	W	T	F	S	S
Drink 8 glasses water	☐	☐	☐	☐	☐	☐	☐
Take my vitamins / supplements	☐	☐	☐	☐	☐	☐	☐
Recorded in my food journal	☐	☐	☐	☐	☐	☐	☐
Measured my weight	☐	☐	☐	☐	☐	☐	☐
Take my electrolytes	☐	☐	☐	☐	☐	☐	☐
Made fat bombs	☐	☐	☐	☐	☐	☐	☐

MEAL PLAN

- _____
- _____
- _____
- _____
- _____
- _____

DID YOU ACCOMPLISH LAST WEEK'S GOALS? IF NOT, WHY?

NEXT WEEK'S GOALS

How I feel today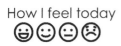

Had cravings today

*"My self-confidence brings out the best in me
and in everyone around me."*

MY GOALS

Date:

FOOD	BREAKFAST	LUNCH	DINNER	SNACKS
	————	————	————	————
	————	————	————	————
	————	————	————	————
	————	————	————	————
	CALORIES :	CALORIES :	CALORIES :	CALORIES :

MACROS	FATS		WEIGHTS & REPS
	CARBS		
	PROTEINS		

FITNESS	WATER INTAKE	CALORIES	SLEEP TIME	WAKE TIME	WEIGHT
MIN / HRS					

NON-SCALE VICTORIES	

How I feel today Had cravings today

😄 😊 😐 😣

"I am reaping the rewards of living life
to the fullest."

MY GOALS

Date:

	BREAKFAST	LUNCH	DINNER	SNACKS
FOOD				
	CALORIES :	CALORIES :	CALORIES :	CALORIES :

			WEIGHTS & REPS
MACROS	**FATS**		
	CARBS		
	PROTEINS		

FITNESS	WATER INTAKE	CALORIES	SLEEP TIME	WAKE TIME	WEIGHT
MIN / HRS	🥛🥛🥛🥛🥛🥛🥛🥛				

	NON-SCALE VICTORIES

How I feel today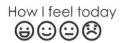

Had cravings today

*"Every day I have the power to choose,
and today I choose to be happy."*

__MY GOALS__

Date:

FOOD	BREAKFAST	LUNCH	DINNER	SNACKS
	————	————	————	————
	————	————	————	————
	————	————	————	————
	————	————	————	————
	CALORIES :	CALORIES :	CALORIES :	CALORIES :

MACROS		WEIGHTS & REPS
FATS		
CARBS		
PROTEINS		

FITNESS	WATER INTAKE	CALORIES	SLEEP TIME	WAKE TIME	WEIGHT
MIN / HRS					

NON-SCALE VICTORIES

How I feel today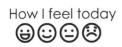

Had cravings today

"Feelings of happiness and serenity come naturally to me."

MY GOALS

Date:

FOOD	BREAKFAST	LUNCH	DINNER	SNACKS
	_____	_____	_____	_____
	_____	_____	_____	_____
	_____	_____	_____	_____
	_____	_____	_____	_____
	CALORIES :	CALORIES :	CALORIES :	CALORIES :

MACROS	FATS		WEIGHTS & REPS
	CARBS		
	PROTEINS		

FITNESS	WATER INTAKE	CALORIES	SLEEP TIME	WAKE TIME	WEIGHT
MIN / HRS					

NON-SCALE VICTORIES

How I feel today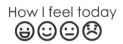

DAY 82

Had cravings today

*"Even in the midst of chaos I can find reasons
to feel happiness and gratitude."*

MY GOALS

Date:

FOOD	BREAKFAST	LUNCH	DINNER	SNACKS
	_____	_____	_____	_____
	_____	_____	_____	_____
	_____	_____	_____	_____
	_____	_____	_____	_____
	CALORIES :	CALORIES :	CALORIES :	CALORIES :

MACROS	FATS		WEIGHTS & REPS
	CARBS		
	PROTEINS		

FITNESS	WATER INTAKE	CALORIES	SLEEP TIME	WAKE TIME	WEIGHT
MIN / HRS					

NON-SCALE VICTORIES

How I feel today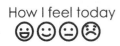

Had cravings today

*"I let go of all resentment and peacefully
welcome the happiness that takes its place."*

MY GOALS

Date:

	BREAKFAST	LUNCH	DINNER	SNACKS
FOOD				
	CALORIES :	CALORIES :	CALORIES :	CALORIES :

MACROS	FATS		WEIGHTS & REPS
	CARBS		
	PROTEINS		

FITNESS	WATER INTAKE	CALORIES	SLEEP TIME	WAKE TIME	WEIGHT
MIN / HRS					

NON-SCALE VICTORIES	

How I feel today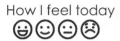

Had cravings today

"Each morning I smile and welcome more happiness into my life."

MY GOALS

Date:

	BREAKFAST	LUNCH	DINNER	SNACKS
FOOD				
	CALORIES :	CALORIES :	CALORIES :	CALORIES :

			WEIGHTS & REPS
MACROS	**FATS**		
	CARBS		
	PROTEINS		

FITNESS	WATER INTAKE	CALORIES	SLEEP TIME	WAKE TIME	WEIGHT
MIN / HRS					

NON-SCALE VICTORIES	

WEEKLY CHECK-IN

CHECK IN

	M	T	W	T	F	S	S
Drink 8 glasses water	☐	☐	☐	☐	☐	☐	☐
Take my vitamins / supplements	☐	☐	☐	☐	☐	☐	☐
Recorded in my food journal	☐	☐	☐	☐	☐	☐	☐
Measured my weight	☐	☐	☐	☐	☐	☐	☐
Take my electrolytes	☐	☐	☐	☐	☐	☐	☐
Made fat bombs	☐	☐	☐	☐	☐	☐	☐

MEAL PLAN

- _____
- _____
- _____

- _____
- _____
- _____

DID YOU ACCOMPLISH LAST WEEK'S GOALS? IF NOT, WHY?

_____

_____

_____

NEXT WEEK'S GOALS

How I feel today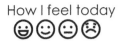

Had cravings today

"Each night I smile and feel deep appreciation
for all the happy experiences of the day."

MY GOALS

Date:

BREAKFAST	LUNCH	DINNER	SNACKS
FOOD			
CALORIES :	CALORIES :	CALORIES :	CALORIES :

MACROS	FATS		WEIGHTS & REPS
	CARBS		
	PROTEINS		

FITNESS	WATER INTAKE	CALORIES	SLEEP TIME	WAKE TIME	WEIGHT
MIN / HRS					

NON-SCALE VICTORIES

How I feel today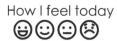

DAY 86

Had cravings today

"Anywhere, any time, I can always choose peace and tranquility."

MY GOALS

Date:

FOOD	BREAKFAST	LUNCH	DINNER	SNACKS
	————	————	————	————
	————	————	————	————
	————	————	————	————
	————	————	————	————
	CALORIES :	CALORIES :	CALORIES :	CALORIES :

MACROS	FATS		WEIGHTS & REPS
	CARBS		
	PROTEINS		

FITNESS	WATER INTAKE	CALORIES	SLEEP TIME	WAKE TIME	WEIGHT
MIN / HRS	🥛🥛🥛🥛🥛🥛🥛🥛				

NON-SCALE VICTORIES	

How I feel today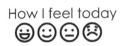

DAY 87

Had cravings today

*"I release all negative thoughts and focus on
positive, productive thinking."*

MY GOALS

Date:

	BREAKFAST	LUNCH	DINNER	SNACKS
FOOD				
	CALORIES :	CALORIES :	CALORIES :	CALORIES :

			WEIGHTS & REPS
MACROS	**FATS**		
	CARBS		
	PROTEINS		

FITNESS	WATER INTAKE	CALORIES	SLEEP TIME	WAKE TIME	WEIGHT
MIN / HRS					

NON-SCALE VICTORIES

How I feel today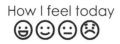

Had cravings today

*"With a simple smile, I have the power
to create happiness for myself and others."*

MY GOALS

Date:

BREAKFAST	LUNCH	DINNER	SNACKS
FOOD			
CALORIES :	CALORIES :	CALORIES :	CALORIES :

MACROS	FATS		WEIGHTS & REPS
	CARBS		
	PROTEINS		

FITNESS	WATER INTAKE	CALORIES	SLEEP TIME	WAKE TIME	WEIGHT
MIN / HRS					

NON-SCALE VICTORIES	

How I feel today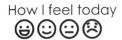

Had cravings today

"Every day I make time for the things that bring happiness to me and my loved ones."

MY GOALS

Date:

FOOD	BREAKFAST	LUNCH	DINNER	SNACKS
	CALORIES :	CALORIES :	CALORIES :	CALORIES :

MACROS	FATS		WEIGHTS & REPS
	CARBS		
	PROTEINS		

FITNESS	WATER INTAKE	CALORIES	SLEEP TIME	WAKE TIME	WEIGHT
MIN / HRS					

NON-SCALE VICTORIES	

How I feel today Had cravings today

DAY 90

" I am grateful for all the people in my life who share their happiness with me."

MY GOALS

Date:

FOOD	BREAKFAST	LUNCH	DINNER	SNACKS
	CALORIES :	CALORIES :	CALORIES :	CALORIES :

MACROS	FATS		WEIGHTS & REPS
	CARBS		
	PROTEINS		

FITNESS	WATER INTAKE	CALORIES	SLEEP TIME	WAKE TIME	WEIGHT
MIN / HRS					

NON-SCALE VICTORIES

WEEKLY CHECK-IN

CHECK IN

	M	T	W	T	F	S	S
Drink 8 glasses water	☐	☐	☐	☐	☐	☐	☐
Take my vitamins / supplements	☐	☐	☐	☐	☐	☐	☐
Recorded in my food journal	☐	☐	☐	☐	☐	☐	☐
Measured my weight	☐	☐	☐	☐	☐	☐	☐
Take my electrolytes	☐	☐	☐	☐	☐	☐	☐
Made fat bombs	☐	☐	☐	☐	☐	☐	☐

MEAL PLAN

- _____
- _____
- _____

- _____
- _____
- _____

DID YOU ACCOMPLISH LAST WEEK'S GOALS? IF NOT, WHY?

_____

_____

_____

NEXT WEEK'S GOALS

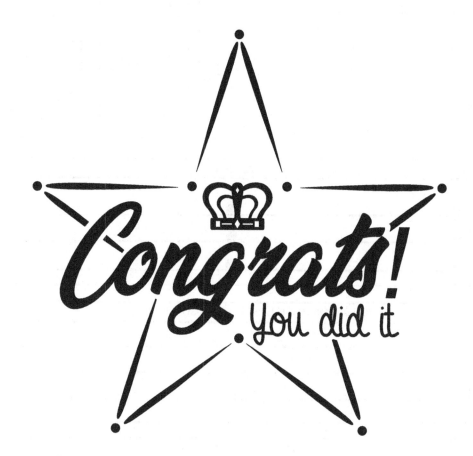

KETO DICTIONARY

Adapted = (see Keto Adapted below)

AS = Artificial Sweetener

BF = Body Fat

BG = Blood Glucose. This means that you're reading how much sugar is there in your body, which is measured by a meter. People suffering from Diabetes test their blood regularly to make sure their sugar levels are optimum.

BMI = Body Mass Index is the ratio between height and weight. It is an established index, whereas the more fat you are, the higher the number. But is controversial because it uses a "one size fits all" method.

BMR = Basal Metabolic Rate = The number of calories your body burns at rest is what your BMR represents

BP = Blood pressure

BPC = Bullet Proof Coffee

Bullet Proof Coffee = I ain't a coffee drinker, but, when you Google it, the best I can tell is it is organically grown "mold free" coffee beans with Unsalted Grass Fed Butter and some kind of oil called (Medium-Chain Triglycerides) are medium chain fatty acids which are extracted from coconut oil. And it has Lauric acid in it. Apparently this coffee tastes really good and gives you Superhuman powers, you never want to eat again, you can leap tall buildings in a single bound and you go into Mars in a few minutes ~ then burning all the remaining fat in your body in a week's time. For newbies: Nope, you don't have to take up coffee drinking to implement the Keto diet.

Carb = Carbohydrate. Any food derived from plants is a carb.

CICO = Calories In Calories Out = the theory states that weight loss is solely from quantitative calorie intake below what a person consumes in energy. The Ketogenic diet proves that the quality or substance that the calorie comes from matters a lot. Once Keto Adapted, the person can lose weight even after the calorie intake is above of what the body uses.

CKD, SKD, TKD = Cyclical Keto Diet, Standard Keto Diet, Targeted Keto Diet, CKD & TKD are Keto Diets for people that do high intensity workouts. Here is a detailed explanation.

CO = Coconut Oil

FA = Fat Adapted, similar to Keto adapted. When one's body derives most of its calories from fat and a very low amount from carbs.

Fat Bombs = Food that is usually sweetened (with lo-carb sweeteners) has a high fat content and low in carbs. Popular ingredients are: coconut oil, cream cheese, butter & cocoa powder.

FODMAPs = Fermentable Oligosaccharides Disaccharides Monosaccharides And Polyols ~ Certain vegetables, fruits and sweeteners that cause digestive problems, in some people, such as: gas, poor digestion, etc. A "low FODMAP" diet would avoid these food items.

Ghee = Clarified butter (high fat). Origin: India, Its butter that has had it's water boiled out of it. All fat. Like concentrated butter.

Glycolysis = A metabolic state that your body is in when your liver turns carbs into glycogen. The glucose is henceforth used by the body as fuel. Glycolysis is the default state your body will be in when it has enough carbs to convert. If the body consumes all of the carbs, your body will then switch over to Ketosis.

Gluconeogenesis = The process whereby the liver converts excess protein into glucose.

H1c or A1C or HA1c = Hemoglobin A1c Test, a test diabetics take that averages the last 3 months of their blood glucose levels. Below 7 is normal.

HF = High Fat

HWC = Heavy Whipping Cream

IBS = Irritable Bowl Syndrome ~ a digestive disorder that commonly causes cramping, abdominal pain, gas, bloating, diarrhea and constipation.

IF = Intermittent Fasting. You eat no food for a minimum of 16 hrs and sometimes even up to a day or two.

IIFYM = If It Fits Your Macros Another position among standard thought, similar to CICO. This definition taken from the web: " Regardless if you like to eat pizza, or boiled chicken breasts, IIFYM teaches us that if you eat less calories than your body requires (while getting adequate protein, carbs, fat and fiber based on your goals and the energy needs of your body) you will lose weight at a steady and predictable rate." Though Many keto'ers disagree with this position.

IR = Insulin Resistance is a condition in which the body produces insulin but doesnt use it effectively. Insulin resistance increases the risk of developing prediabetes and type 2 diabetes.

KCKO = Keep Calm Keto On! A phrase to ensourage someone their KETO journey.

Keto = abbreviated version of the word: Ketogenic
Ketoacidosis = Not to be confused with ketosis. Ketoacidosis is a rare condition found in diabetics (Usually T1) and severe alcoholics, leading up to a severe excess of ketones. In the case of diabetics, it is mainly because the diabetes is uncontrolled and the body is producing no insulin. Normal ketogenic ketone levels range from .5 mmol/L (a measurement of ketone concentration in the blood) to 3.5 mmol/L. Ketoacidosis is a concentration usually in excess of 15 mmol/L.

Keto Adapted = When your body is in the ketosis state for 2 to 4 weeks, your body will move into metabolic state where it builds enzymes and hormones that are adapted to burn fat more efficiently. This is the goal of the Keto diet. This is the short definition.

Keto Flu = On the induction phase of the Keto diet, your body may give you some "flu like" symptoms. If you cut the carbs drastically your body has to adjust hormonally for burning fat. A lot of the flu comes from an electrolyte deficiency you will get, because your liver will start dumping electrolytes after it switches over to producing fatty acids. Here is a much more comprehensive explanation for Keto flu.

Ketogenic Diet = Low Carb, High Fat, Medium Protein diet

Keto Sub Groups = There are different types of Ketogenic diets, too numerous to list here.

Ketosis = A metabolic state that your body is in, when the liver turns fat into fatty acids called ketones. The ketones then are used by the body as fuel. This state is induced by water fasting or by limiting your diet to a very small amount of carbs per day.

Keto'ers = Those that believe or practice the Ketogenic lifestyle.

Keto Rash = An itchy rash that develops after starting a Ketogenic diet. This is probably a candida die off. After the die off, the liver cannot clean out the endotoxins produced by the die off, resulting in a rash. The rash will go away eventually, do not stop the diet.

Kryptonite Food = Low carb high fat food that tastes so good, you can't stop eating it. You eat too many calories of it. Some common kryptonite foods may include: Bacon, nuts or other tree pecans, etc.

LCHF = Low Carb High Fat (Ketogenic diet)
LC or LCD = Lo Carb or Low Carb Diet
LBM = Lean Body Mass The weight of your body minus essential fats.
Locavore = a person whose diet consists only or principally of locally grown or produced food.

Low FODMAP Diet = Fermentable Oligo-Di-Monosaccharides and Polyols

This group of people have digestive problems when eating certain kinds of sugars that can cause bloating, constipation, etc. Some also have inflammatory bowel disease. You have to restrict consumption of fructose, fructans, lactose, galactans, and other polyols sugars found in certain fruits and zero-calorie sweeteners.

Macros = Macronutrients, your diet ratio between: Carbs, Fat & Protein. These three food components are the "fuel" for your body. They are expressed in terms of percentages of each in relation to your diet in calories. The most popular ratio for Keto is: 75% Fat, 20% protein & 5% carbs..

MCT = Medium Chain Triglycerides. Fatty acids in many oils and milk. A very healthy oil. Usually associated with coconut oil.

MFP = MyFitnessPal

Micros = Micronutrients small amounts of minerals or vitamins that belong in our daily diet to promote healthy living. There are minimums established, but some believe their guidelines are not correct or there isn't a "one-size-fits-all" approach to the amounts recommended. The micronutrients are measured in milligrams.

MUFA = Mono-Unsaturated Fatty Acid. This is a good fat. Here is a better definition.

NK = Nutritional Ketosis, see "Keto Adapted"
NSV = Non-scale Victory These are benefits derived from the Ketogenic way of living that are not connected to weight loss. These could be, improved blood tests, better fitting clothes, feeling better, clearer mind, less sickness, etc.

OWL or Atkins OWL = Ongoing Weight Loss

Paleo, Paleo diet, Paleolithic, Caveman diet = Another diet regime that you do not eat processed foods like grains, vegetable & grain oils, legumes, dairy and sugar. It promotes eating food available that is found wild in nature, berries, nuts, usually organically grown. It parallels the Keto diet, in that, you avoid grains, highly processed high carb starchy foods.

PCOS = PolyCystic Ovary Syndrome

PISS = Post-Induction Stall Syndrome: A couple weeks after being on the diet and before you are "adapted" you will find that water and glycogen find a new balance and this causes a stall or even weight gain, which lasts for a week or two. Relax, PISS is both normal and temporary.

PSMF = Protein-Sparing Modified Fast. PSMF is a lo-carb, lo-fat, lo-calorie diet. Rapid weight loss. A long-term PSMF diet undertaken carelessly and without the care of a physician may lead to serious health risks.

PT = Physical Therapy (being heavy can injure you and you may need this occasionally)

PUFA = Polyunsaturated Fatty Acid. Bad fats with excessive levels of Omega-6s which can cause damaging inflammation, particularly when subjected to high temperatures, like in cooking. Example: canola oil, vegetable oil and other grain oils (basically oils that require massive processing to obtain.)

RDA = Recommended Daily Allowance. Usually associated with how much minerals and vitamins you should take. Set by the government.

SA = Sugar Alcohols Sweeteners that are carb free, and usually end with the letters, "ol". For example: Erythritol, Xylitol, Sorbitol, Mannitol to name a few.

S.A.D. or SAD = Standard American Diet (Low sodium, Low Fat, High Carb diet) This diet has been blamed for the current epidemic of overweight, metabloic syndrome, morbidly obese, insuline resistant population that is stressing out the medical system. This diet was institututed and promulgated in the 70's by the U.S. government and exported to most of the rest of the world (with a similar effect on foreign populations.)

Scraping = If you have to eat a pizza, you "scrape" all the toppings off (ditch the crust) to keep it a low carb meal.

TDEE = Total Daily Energy Expenditure = TDEE is the amount calories your body burns in a 24 hour period, sleeping, working, exercising, playing and even digesting food! calculator

T2D or T2 or TII or T1 = Type 2 Diabetic or Type 2 Diabetes or Type 1 diabetic

TLDR or TL;DR = Too long, don't read!

WOE = Way Of Eating

WOL = Way of Life ~ in the context of nutrition: to chose a method of eating consistantly and routinely for the rest of your life ~ as opposed to a temporary diet.

YMMV = Your Mileage May Vary ~ a term to explain that works for the original poster, may not work as well for you.

Join our Keep Calm Keto On Facebook Group
to receive a free kindle copy of your
Keto On Journal
(only for kindle unlimited members)
and other great deals and promotions:

https://www.facebook.com/groups/KeepCalmKetoOn/

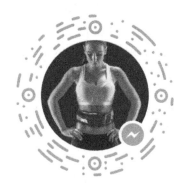

Made in the USA
Middletown, DE
04 January 2020